About This Book

Tobacco consumption is the chief avoidable cause of death in our society, yet millions of people continue to smoke and chew tobacco. This book explains how tobacco use can lead to:

- stained teeth and other problems with appearance
- bad breath
- a decrease in the senses of smell and taste
- facial wrinkling
- the development of tartar (calculus)
- changes in periodontal structures (gums and supporting bone)
- impaired wound healing with dental therapy, such as implants
- a variety of other oral conditions including dental abrasion, hairy tongue, smoker's palate, leukoplakia, chronic sinusitis, and oral cancer.

The book also explains how to achieve a healthier and longer life by stopping tobacco use, including:

- developing a tobacco-free lifestyle
- the health benefits of quitting
- understanding addiction
- becoming an ex-tobacco user
- choosing a cessation program
- tips for staying tobacco free

For more detailed information on any of these subjects, ask your dentist or hygienist.

Why Is Tobacco So Harmful?

You may have heard about some of the negative effects of tobacco, such as lung cancer, heart disease, and respiratory diseases, but tobacco use also has significant effects on your mouth and teeth that you may not know about.

All forms of tobacco can negatively affect your mouth. The tobacco in cigarettes, cigars, and pipes contains over 4,000 harmful chemicals and gases, and 50 of these are cancer-producing. Likewise, smokeless (chewing) tobacco has about 3,000 chemicals, and 28 of these are carcinogenic (can cause cancer). Many of these compounds act directly as irritants and poisons (toxins) to mouth tissues.

The most direct negative effect on the mouth is chemical in nature. However, oral tissue damage also occurs when the lining of the mouth is heated and dried out during smoking. Also, during snuff dipping or tobacco chewing, a pinch of spit tobacco or a "chaw" of leaf or plug tobacco is placed directly against the oral soft tissues, bathing the entire mouth in tobacco juice.

Contact with the irritating and dangerous chemicals produced by all forms of tobacco can cause extensive oral damage within a relatively short period.

A Healthy, Tobacco-Free Mouth

This is a healthy tobacco-free mouth with no signs of dental disease. The breath is nonoffensive; the tongue is pink, clean, and uncoated; and the teeth are unstained by tobacco tars. The gum tissues surrounding the teeth are firm, pink, and do not bleed.

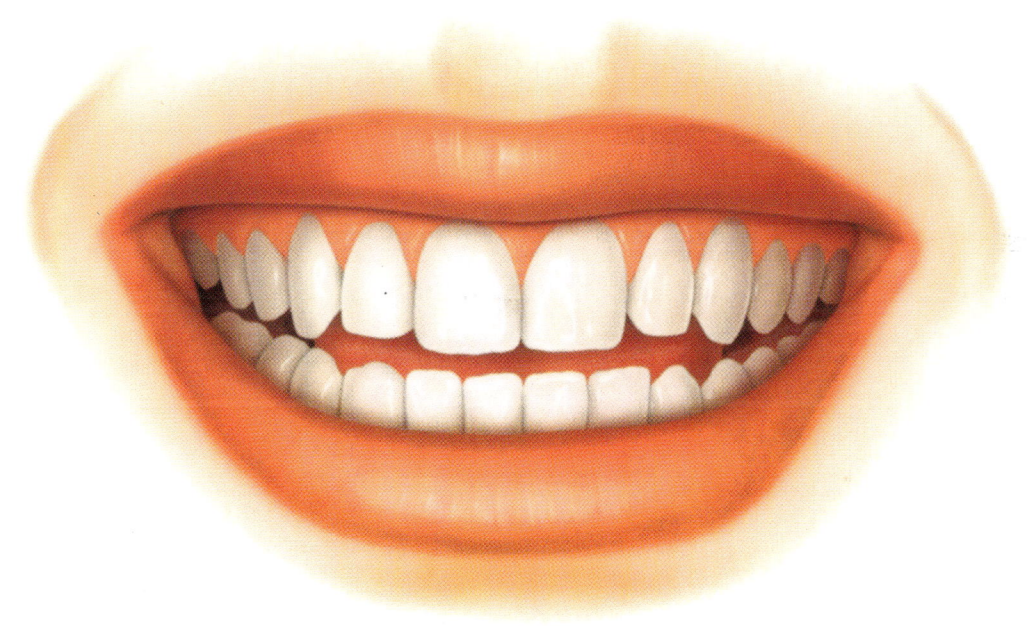

Premature Wrinkling

Tobacco advertisements try to convince you that smoking will make you appear glamorous, attractive, and youthful. Although normal aging causes some facial wrinkling, smoking speeds up this process, especially around the mouth, eyes, and neck. This condition, sometimes called "smoker's face" occurs most often in those who have smoked cigarettes for 20 years or more.

"Smoker's Face"

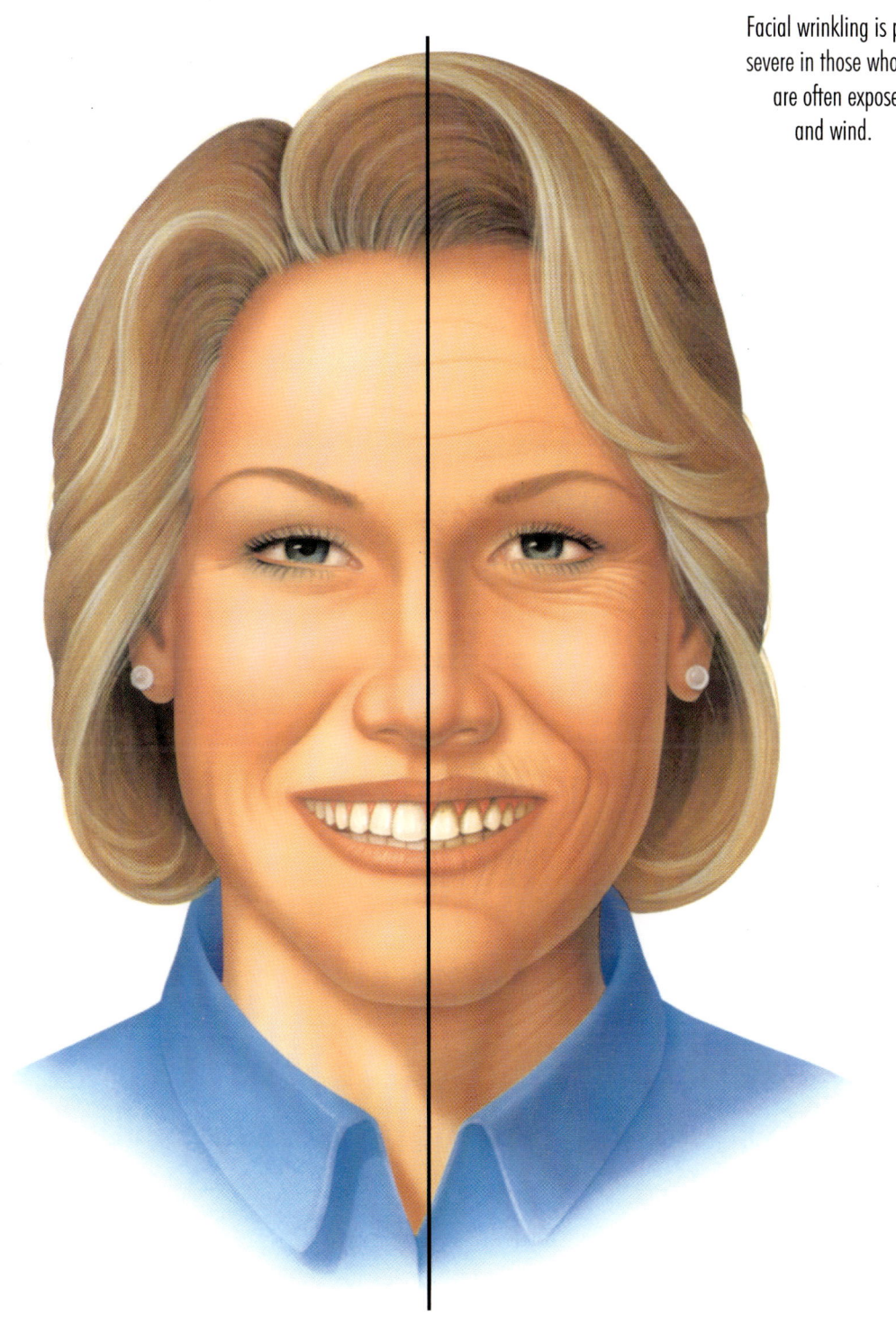

Facial wrinkling is particularly severe in those who smoke and are often exposed to sunlight and wind.

Tobacco Stains

Smokers have more brown and black stains on their teeth, in their fillings, and or their dentures than nonsmokers. A dental professional may be able to remove these unsightly discolorations, but sometimes the stains penetrate tooth structures and dental materials deeply. This makes complete removal impossible, especially if the roots of the teeth are exposed, that is, if the gums have pulled away from the teeth, or receded.

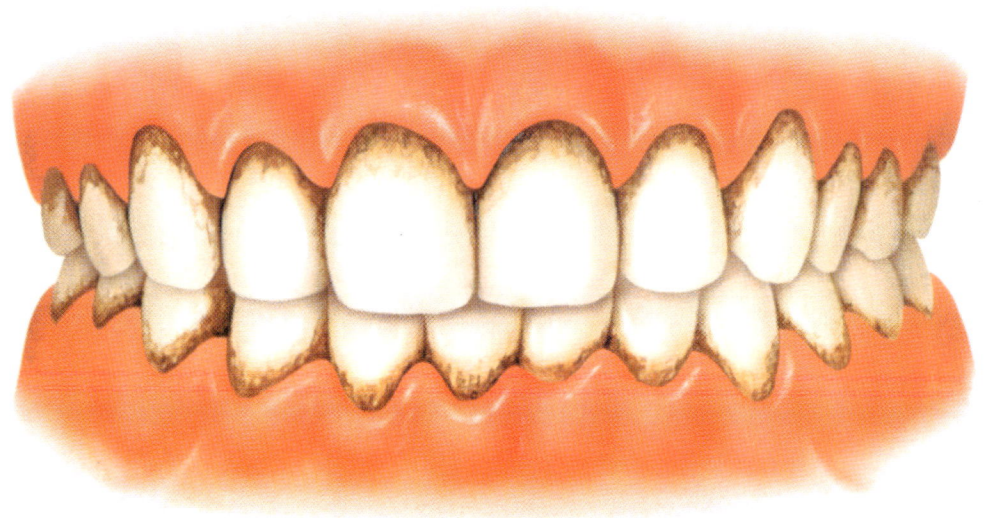

All forms of tobacco stain teeth, dentures, and filling materials, and cause a harmful buildup of dental calculus (tartar). Tobacco also produces unpleasant breath odor (halitosis).

Bad Breath, Tobacco Stains, and Calculus

Tobacco-associated bad breath is directly related to the odor intensity of the type of tobacco that is used. Cigar and pipe tobaccos are stronger than cigarette tobacco. They contain a larger amount of sulfur—the same chemical that you smell when eggs rot. That's why smoking them produces stronger offensive breath.

Proper oral cleaning and quitting tobacco use significantly reduce bad breath, staining, and tartar buildup.

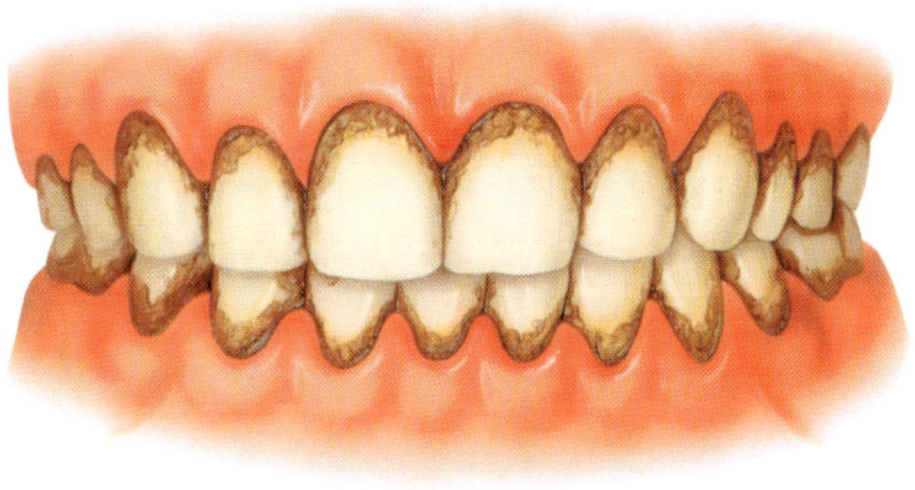

Here are the results of tobacco use: stained teeth and a buildup of dental calculus (tartar).

Chemical Erosion Produced by Breath Mints

To mask tobacco-related bad breath, some people use mouth-washes, chewing gum, candy, or breath mints. Habitually sucking candy or mints, which contain sugar and often citric acid, can cause severe chemical erosion. The tooth surface (enamel) gradually erodes, often leading to dental decay.

Here are the results of attempting to cover up bad breath by habitually sucking candy or mints.

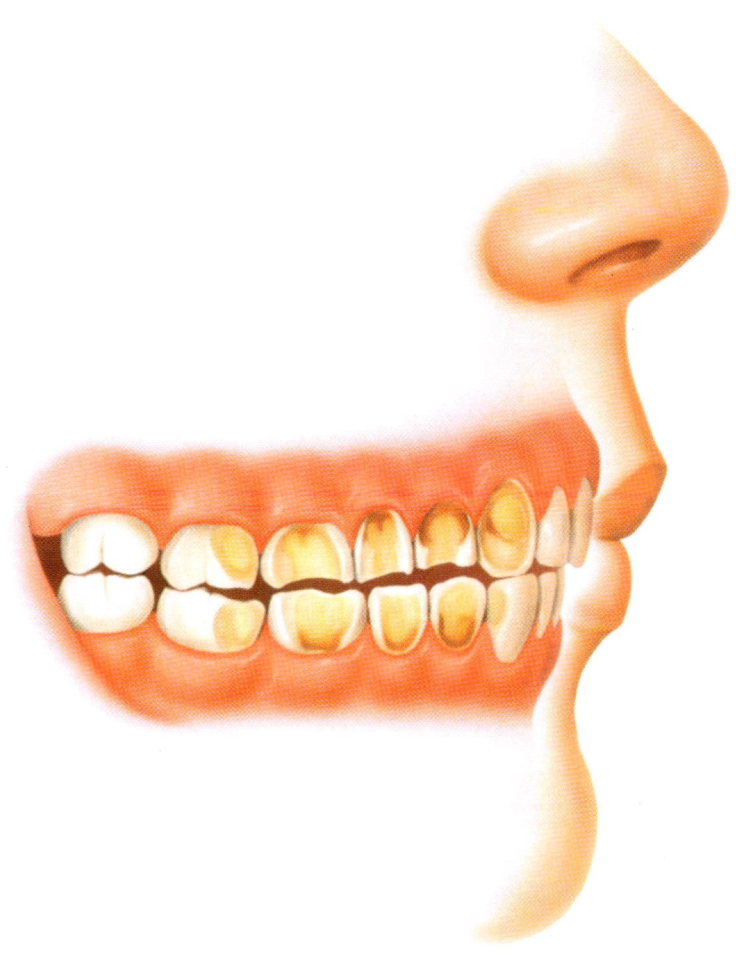

Both adult and teenage smokers have higher levels of tartar formation than nonsmokers. This hard, mineralized deposit builds up both above and below the gumline and must be removed by a dental professional. The more someone smokes, the greater the buildup of calculus. Calculus formation decreases after quitting.

Tartar (Calculus) Formation

Calculus buildup makes it much easier for plaque to stick to your teeth in such a way that you cannot remove it by brusing and flossing. Plaque is full of bacteria that cause gum disease and cavities.

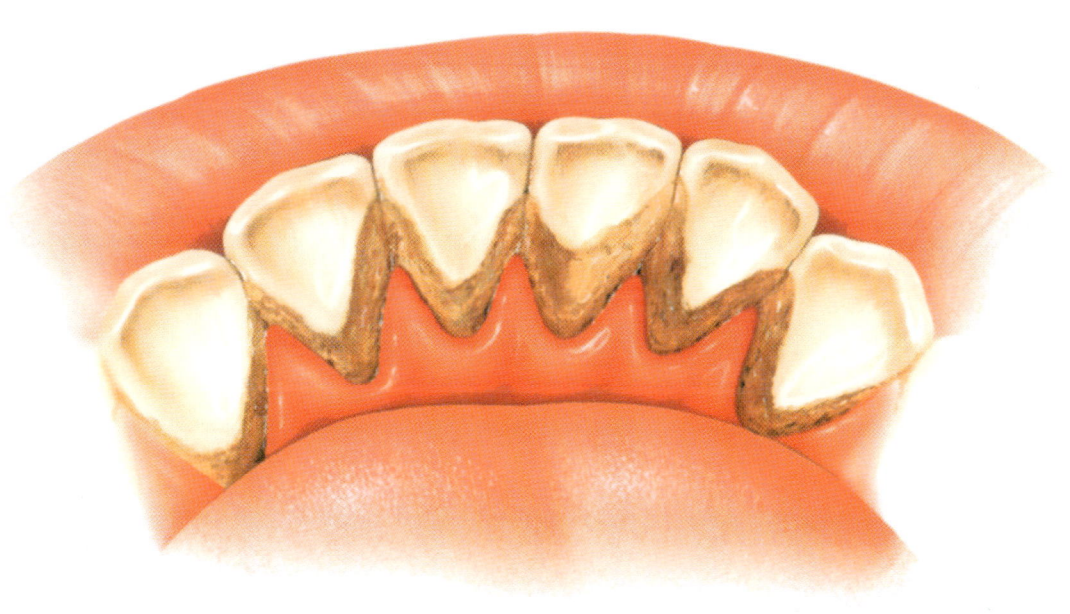

Tooth Wear

Tooth wear, or abrasion, occurs when tooth structures are worn away through an abnormal mechanical or frictional process. Pipe smokers and long-term smokeless tobacco users are prone to wear on the biting edges of their teeth, which are often worn flat.

Gritty sand substances that occur naturally in smokeless tobacco cause these drastic wear patterns. The tiny particles of sand act like an emery board, gradually filing down tooth surfaces over time.

Pipe smokers often develop wear on their teeth from holding the pipestem in the same place in the mouth. When this abrasive activity causes the softer part of the tooth (called dentin) to become exposed, deep tobacco-related staining may occur.

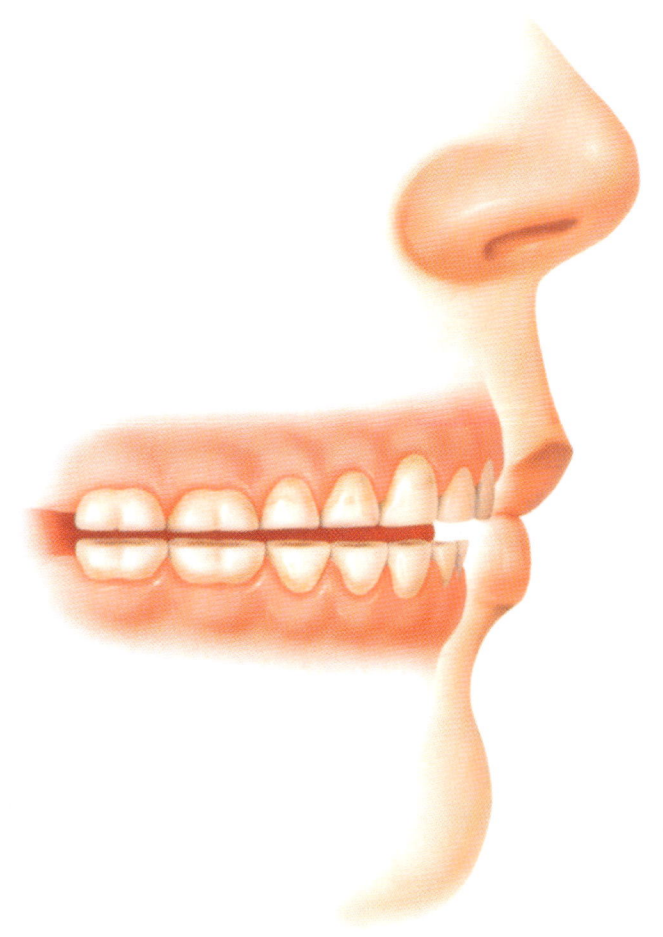

Periodontal (Gum) Disease

Tobacco users, especially cigarette smokers, are more prone to develop severe periodontal (gum) diseases than nonsmokers. Gum disease can involve bone loss around the teeth, deeper gaps between the teeth and gums, loose teeth, and eventually tooth loss. The more tobacco used, and the longer it is used, the greater the destruction of the tissues around the affected teeth. These effects are the same in men and women.

One symptom of gum disease is bleeding around the gums. But due to the chemical effects of tobacco, a smoker's gums may not bleed readily, even when disease is present. If there is no bleeding, the patient may be unaware of the condition and not seek treatment, allowing the disease to progress rapidly.

Quitting smoking can significantly slow the development of gum disease and reduce the rate of destructive bone and tooth loss.

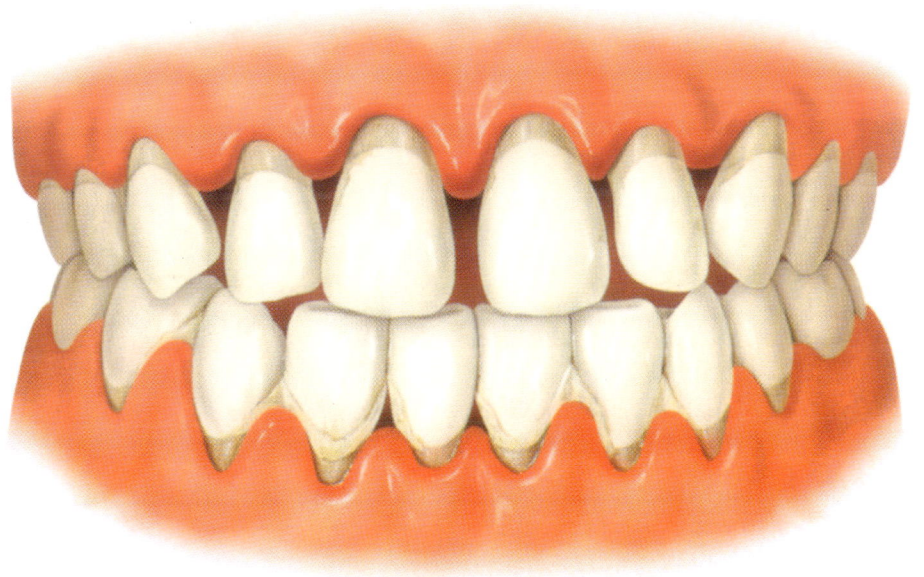

Trench Mouth

A severe, recurrent, painful infection of the gums around and between the teeth is known as trench mouth, acute necrotizing gingivitis, or Vincent's disease. It produces bleeding, ulcerated gums, excessive saliva, and extremely offensive breath. Those who smoke ten or more cigrattes per day have a much greater chance of developing this infection than those who don't smoke. Poor oral hygiene, poor nutrition, and stress are linked to the development of this disease. This condition is treatable, but may recur, especially with continued smoking.

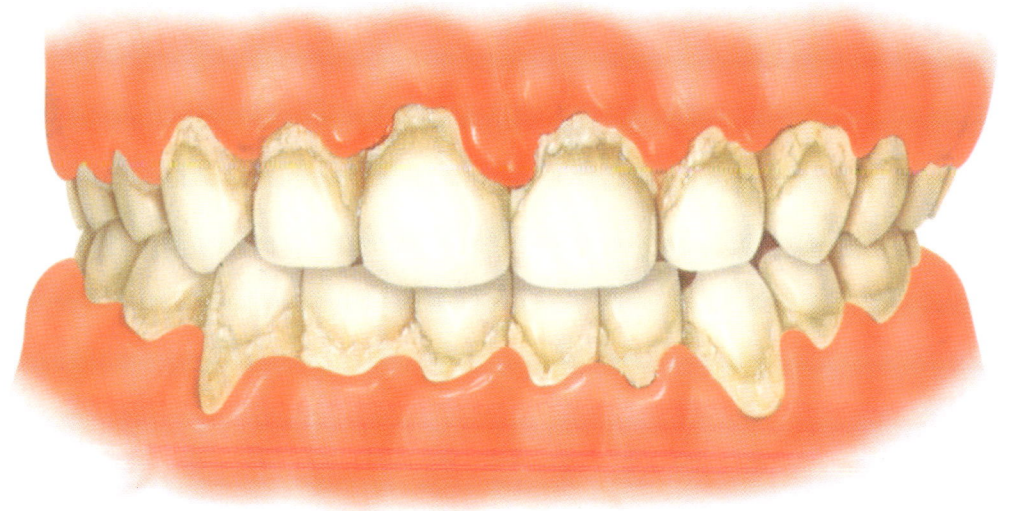

Smoker's Palate

This condition often develops in the mouths of heavy pipe, cigarette, and cigar smokers. The roof of the mouth typically resembles a cobblestone street, with many white, slightly raised bumps with red spots in the center.

Smoker's palate usually disappears in a few weeks after smoking has been discontinued.

Although most cases of smoker's palate are not serious, severe forms can progress to oral cancer.

Smoker's palate shown in a heavy pipe smoker.

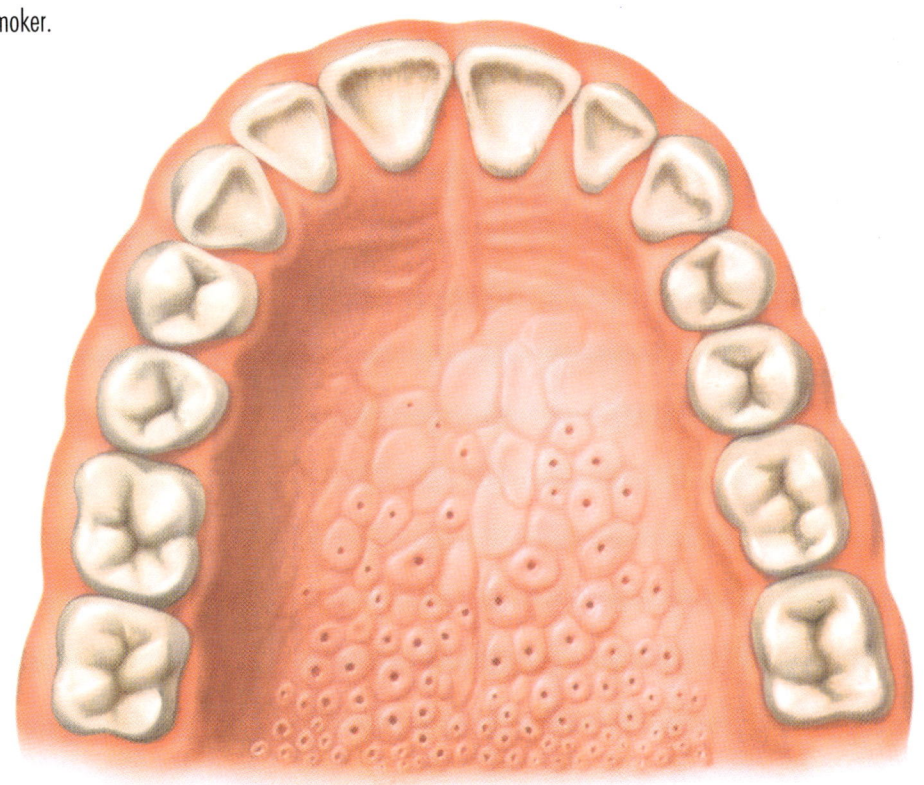

Hairy Tongue

Heavy cigarette smoking can produce an unsightly overgrowth of the tiny projections on the tongue's surface (called papilla). This yellowish white, brown, or black, furlike coating resembles hair. Eventually, germs and food debris become trapped between these projections and can cause a burning sensation on the tongue. Extremely bad breath also accompanies hairy tongue.

To correct this condition, hairy tongue suffers should stop using tobacco and brush or gently scrape their tongues daily.

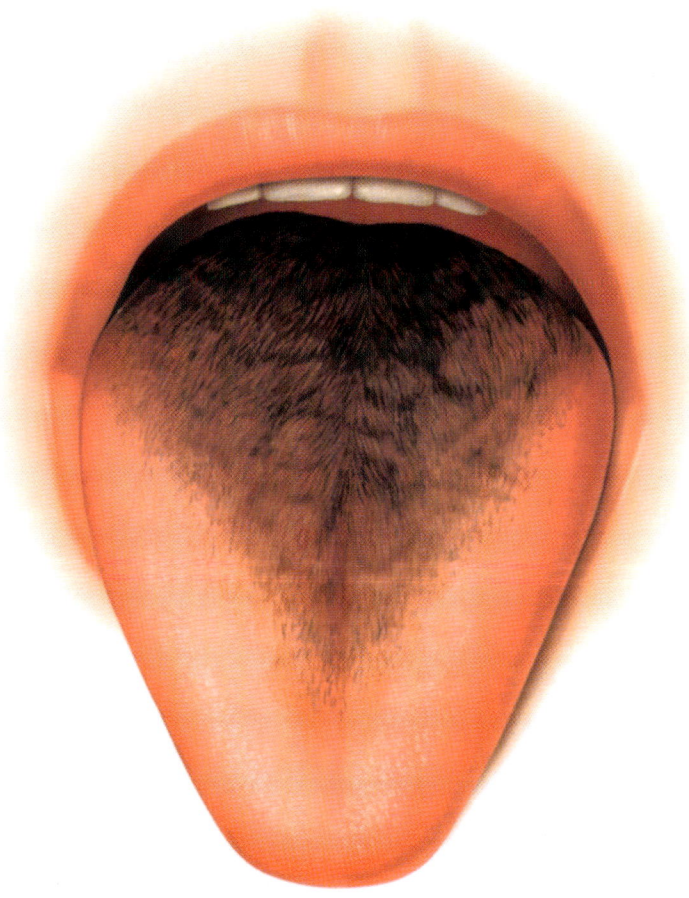

Chronic sinusitis is an inflammation of the tissues lining the sinus cavities. The condition affects millions of people. Those who are especially sensitive to tobacco smoke develop swelling in their nasal membranes. The swelling blocks sinus openings and causes pain. Sinusitis occurs more frequently among smokers than nonsmokers, and is often significantly reduced when smoking is discontinued. Sinus discomfort can often mimic the pain of a toothache.

Chronic Sinus Infections

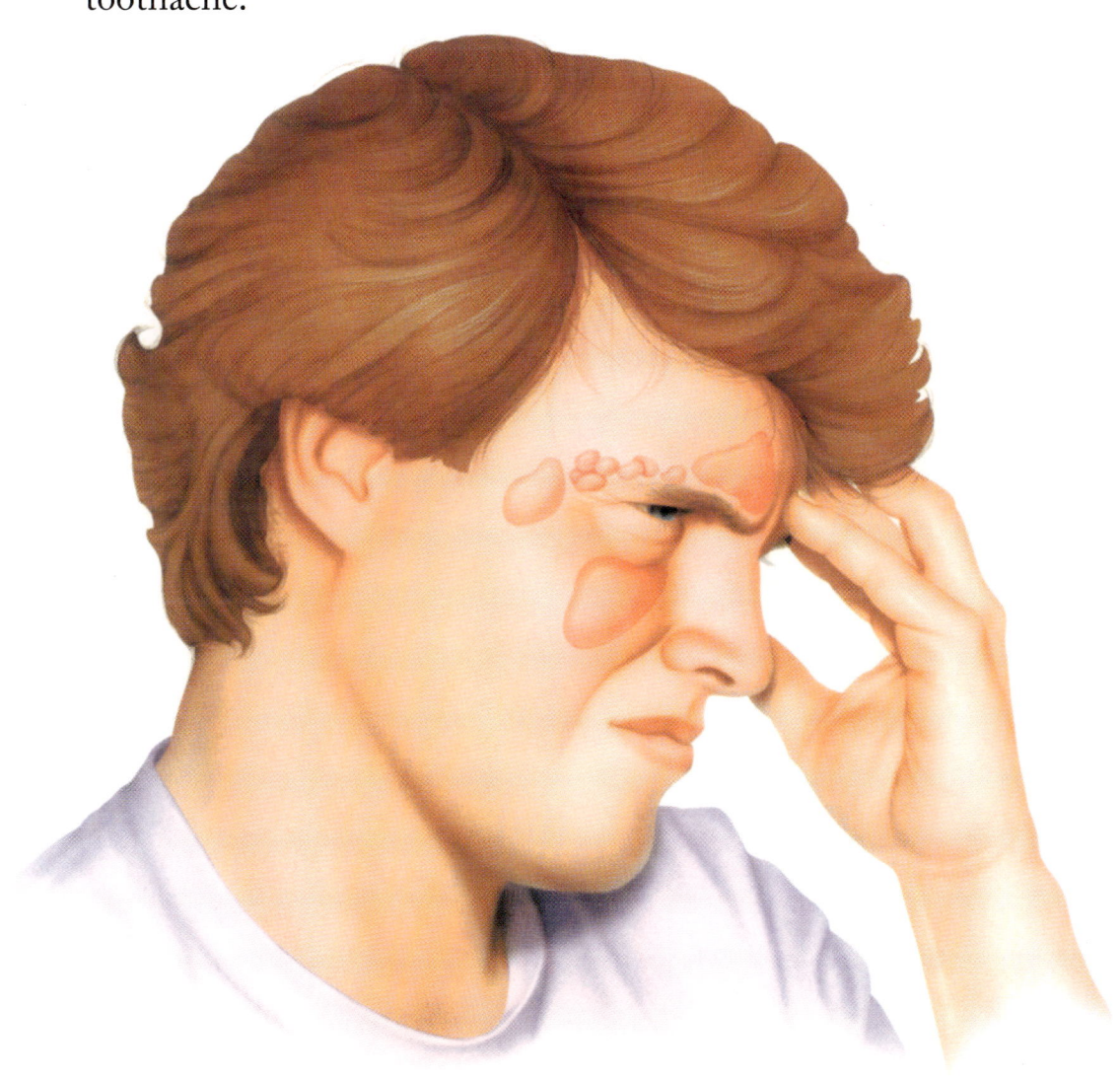

Tobacco Use Impairs Wound Healing

Tobacco use (especially cigarette smoking) may delay wound healing in individuals who have mouth infections or oral ulcers. It can also impair healing in those who have had recent tooth extractions, gum surgery, bone grafting procedures, or implant placement.

There are over 4,000 known gases and chemicals in tobacco smoke, and many of these act directly on mouth tissues. The nicotine in your body constricts your blood vessels, causing them to become narrower. This makes it much more difficult for oxygen-rich blood to reach a wound. Oxygen acts as "food" for wounded tissues, fueling the healing process. If the oxygen supply is limited, the wound will not heal as it should.

Continued tobacco use hampers the healing process after any type of oral surgery.

Narrowed blood vessels make it difficult for oxygen-rich blood to reach a wound.

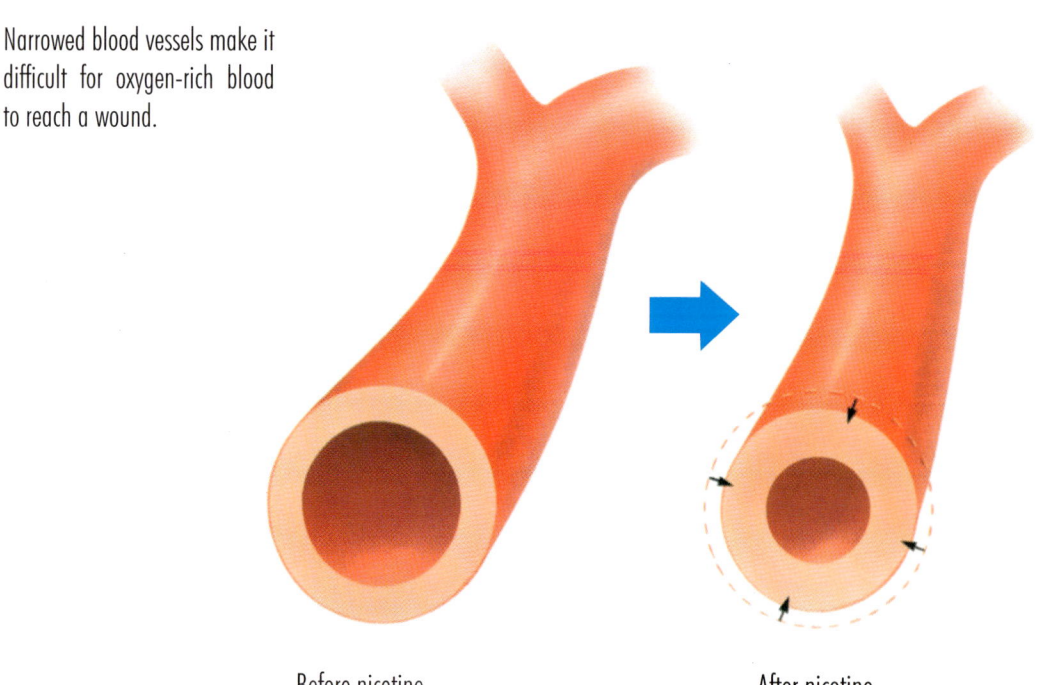

Before nicotine   After nicotine

Dental Implants and Tobacco

Dental implants are devices that are placed in the bone underneath the gums to replace missing teeth. Artificial teeth are later attached to the implants. Implant placement is a surgical procedure, and the tissue around the implant must heal before the artificial tooth can be attached.

Cigarette smoking has been found to be a major factor in the failure of dental implants due to impaired would healing, as described on the previous page. If you smoke, the tissue around a dental implant may not heal effectively and treatment may be compromised. By quitting tobacco use four weeks before implant placement, and permanently after implant placement, a smoker can reduce and control these damaging effects.

After healing, keeping the implant clean is extremely important. This may be more difficult for a smoker.

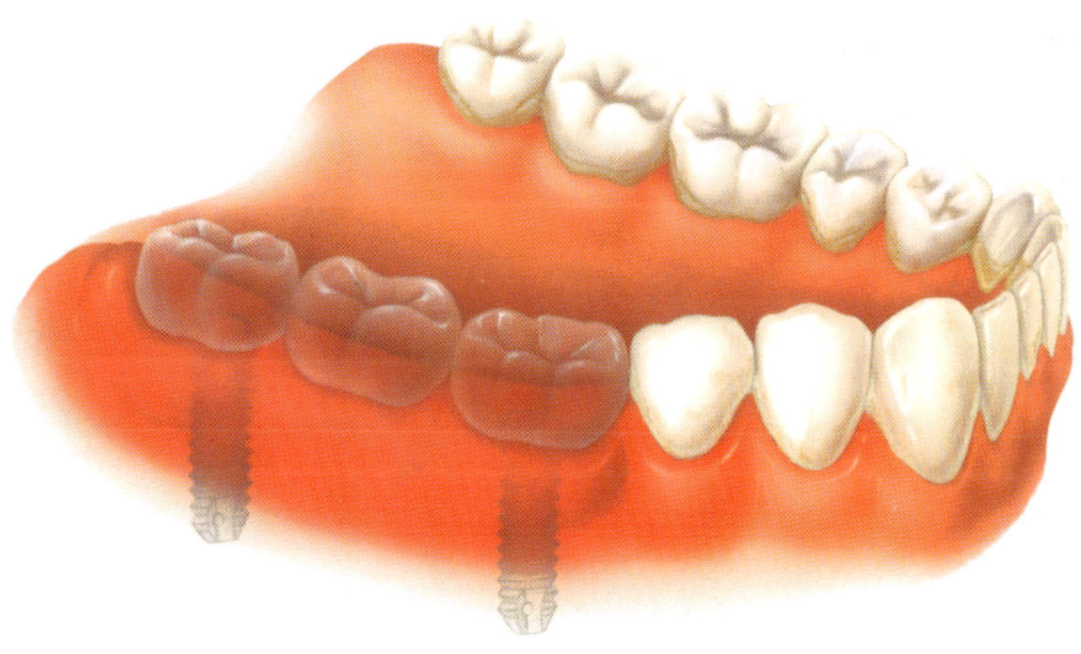

17

Tobacco White Patch (Leukoplakia)

Leukoplakia, a white patch, is most commonly seen inside the cheeks of 50- to 70-year-old men. It is often related to other oral conditions such as badly fitting dentures, broken teeth, or the effects of tobacco. Although it is not seen exclusively in tobacco users, it has been definitely associated with both smoking and smokeless tobacco use.

Leukoplakias of the mouth are considered to be precancerous, which means they could progress to cancer. These white patches may disappear completely within a matter of weeks after tobacco use is discontinued.

To rule out cancer, your dentist may need to examine the white patch further by taking a tiny sample (called a biopsy) or referring you to a pathologist or oral surgeon.

Cigar smoking, which is increasing among men and women, is not a safe alternative to cigarettes or smokeless tobacco. It is strongly associated with the development of oral leukoplakia.

Here leukoplakia is shown in the corner of the mouth, where a cigar smoker would habitually hold a lit— or unlit—cigar.

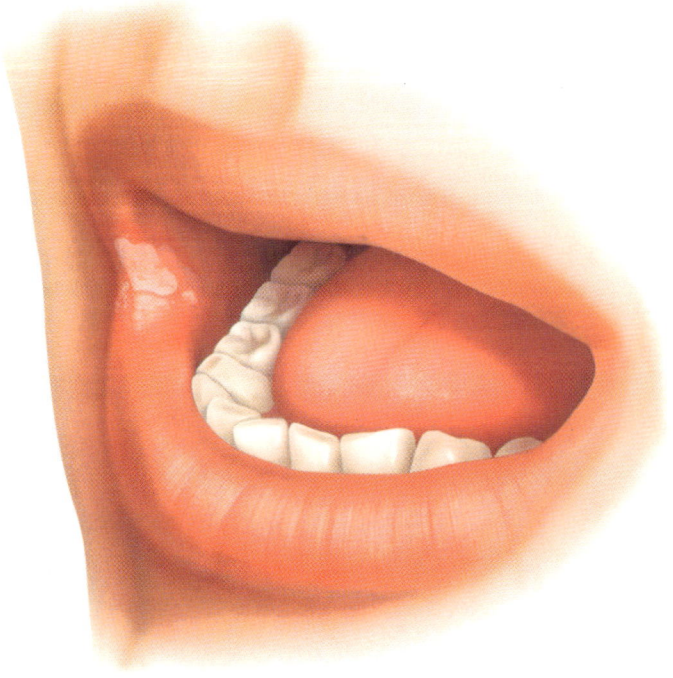

Oral Cancer

Tobacco damages the soft tissues in your mouth and can lead to mouth cancer. Sometimes, even relatively harmless-looking red or white patches in the mouth can become cancerous. The most common sites for mouth cancers are the lip, cheek, an tongue.

The risk of developing cancer of the mouth, larynx, pharynx, and esophagus is significantly higher for smokers than for nonsmokers. About 30,000 people are diagnosed and treated for oral cancer each year in the United States. Virtually all of these victims have used tobacco in some form. Any form of smoking combined with drinking alcohol on a regular basis increases the rate of head and neck cancer. In adults who do not smoke or drink, cancer of the mouth and throat almost never occur. Smoking and drinking alcohol work together to increase the possibility of developing oral cancer. Five years after quitting, a former smoker's risk of developing a new cancer of the mouth or throat reduces by half; the risks continue to decrease as time goes on.

Tobacco white patch, next to an early, innocent-appearing cancer of the lower lip (arrow).

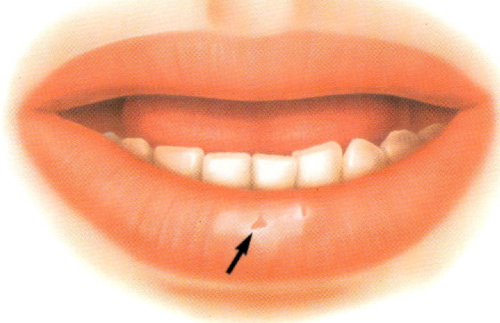

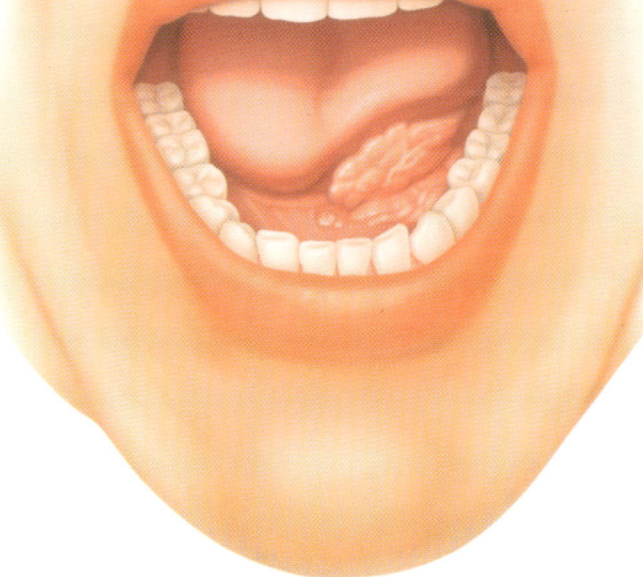

An advanced tobacco-related cancer of the tongue and floor of the mouth, such as the one shown here, can be fatal.

What Is Smokeless Tobacco?

Smokeless tobacco comes in several different forms and has many different names, including dip, chaw, snuff, plug, pinch, and spit tobacco. It contains about 3,000 chemicals, 28 of which can cause cancer, and is every bit as addictive as cigarette tobacco. One pinch or quid of smokeless tobacco contains the same amount of nicotine as 2.5 cigarettes.

Snuff dippers place a pinch of powdered tobacco (sold in cans or individual packets) between their cheek and gum; tobacco chewers place leaf tobacco (in a pouch) or plug tobacco (in brick form) between the cheek and gum. Any form of smokeless tobacco can seriously harm your dental health.

Remember: Using smokeless tobacco is not a safe alternative to smoking.

Warning signals: *If you use smokeless tobacco, pull back your lips and cheeks—look closely at the area where you hold your tobacco. Your teeth and gums may show that damage is occurring. If you see a white patch, a red sore that doesn't heal, or a lump on your cheek, tongue, or gums, see your hygienist or dentist immediately.*

Snuff Dipper's Patch and Gum Recession

A snuff dipper's patch often looks like the wrinkled hide of an elephant. It occurs underneath the lip, and can result in severe gum loss (recession) and bone loss around affected teeth. These dramatic changes can develop after using smokeless tobacco for only a few months. Quitting often makes the whitish color and wrinkling go away, but damage to the gum tissues and bone will remain.

Gum recession commonly occurs in the area next to the spot where a smokeless tobacco quid is held. About one-half of users experience recession, or the "skin pulling away from the teeth." This condition can become quite severe, and lead to tooth loss as the supporting bone around the tooth is destroyed.

Severe bone and gum tissue loss occurs under the smokeless tobacco quid.

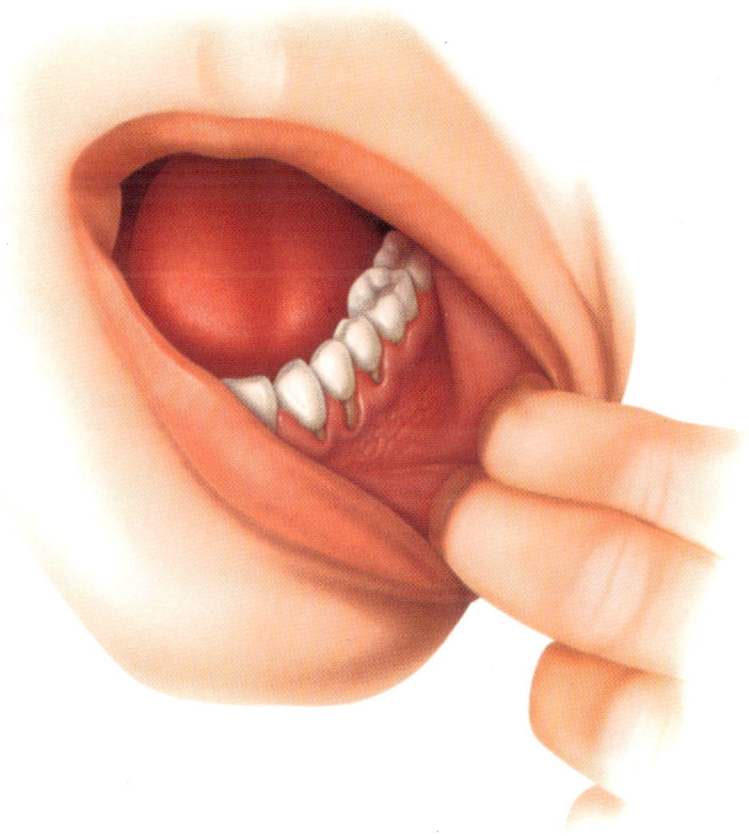

Leukoplakia Caused by Chewing Tobacco

Some well-known athletes have developed tobacco chewing into an art form. But here is the result—leukoplakia, which appears as thickened bands of tissue with white and red furrows.

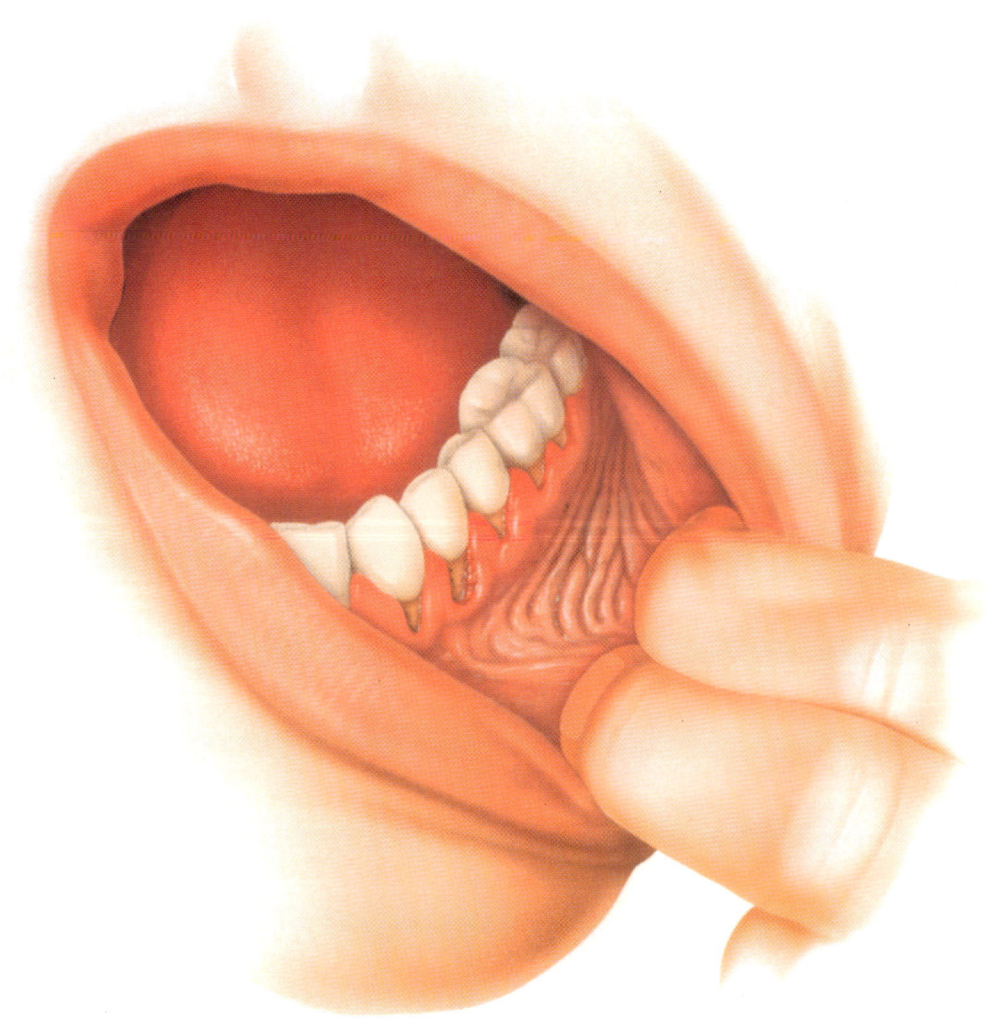

Smokeless Tobacco and Orthodontics

Smokeless tobacco users who wear braces or other fixed orthodontic appliances hold the quid closely against their teeth. Visible clumps of tobacco become packed into and around the braces. As a result, the gums recede and severe root exposure can occur within relatively short time. The resulting root exposure is permanent—it will not repair itself when the braces are removed. Tobacco may also cause severe stains on the teeth around brackets.

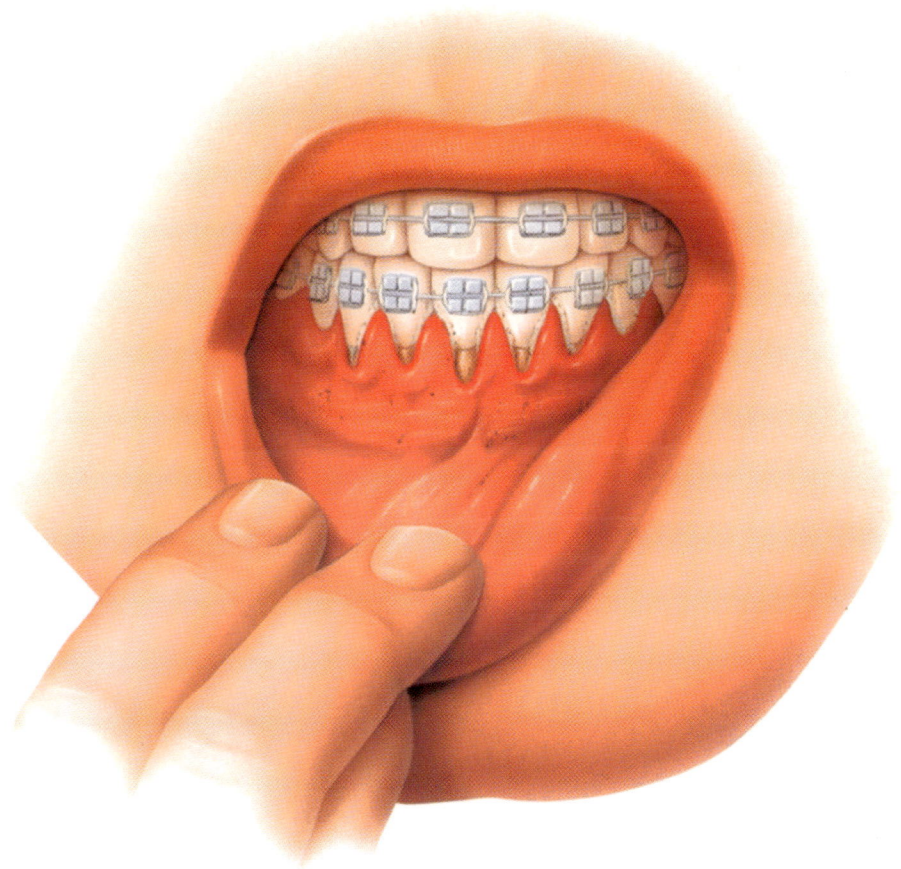

Developing a Tobacco-Free Lifestyle

This section explains the process of tobacco cessation, including the benefits of quitting, understanding addiction, and some information about choosing a cessation program.

Why Quit?

We have shown you the effects of tobacco use on your oral health. Most people know that many life-threatening conditions are related to continued tobacco use, such as:

- cancers of the lung, mouth, larynx, and urinary tract
- hardening of the arteries, coronary heart disease, and stroke

- asthma, bronchitis, and emphysema

Some long-term tobacco users may believe that it is too late for them to stop because they have already done so much damage to their bodies. However, most of the physical effects of tobacco use are reversible— it's never too late to quit.

It is important to understand the general nature of addiction, and determine the degree of your individual tobacco dependency. By completing the two self-tests the Fagerström Test for Nicotine Dependence and the Smoker's (Horn) Self-Test) you can determine your degree of addiction to tobacco.

Nicotine addiction can be viewed as a three-linked chain of enslavement: physical dependence (the central link); and psychological considerations and social factors (the adjoining links).

Understanding Addiction

Addiction: a slavish physical and/or emotional dependence on a harmful, habit-forming substance and/or behaviour.

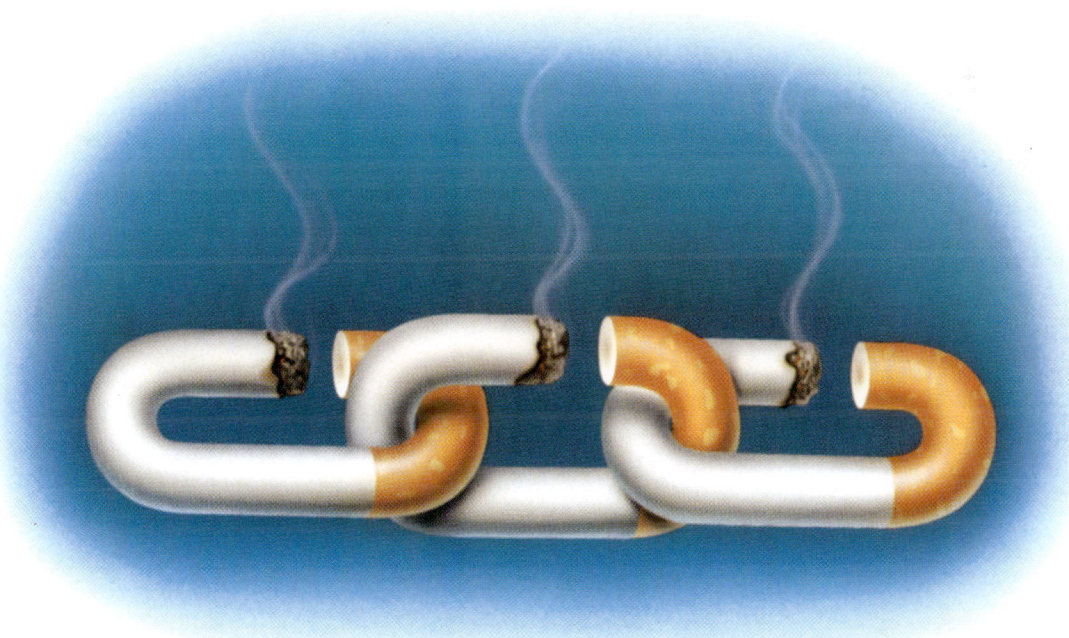

Psychological
considerations

Physical
dependence

Social
factors

The Health Benefits of Quitting

When you stop using tobacco, your body immediately begins to heal in the following ways:

Within 5 minutes	• Oxygen has become more available to your heart muscles
Within 20 minutes	• your pulse and blood pressure levels have returned to normal • the temperature of your hands and feet have risen Within 8 hours
Within 8 minutes	• your blood platelets are less likely to clump, and thereby block your arteries • the carbon monoxide in your blood has been reduced to a normal level
Within 24 minutes	• your risk of having a heart attack has decreased significantly • your physical endurance and energy have increased
Within 48 hours	• your sense of taste, smell, and food enjoyment have improved • the stale smoke odors on your breath and body have disappeared
Within 2 weeks	• your lung function has increased, and you can breathe more easily • your body's ability to metabolize medications has returned to normal • your nagging cough has disappeared
Within 3 months	• your rate of gum disease development has slowed down significantly • your possibility of having a stroke has decreased to the level of a nonsmoker • the "bad lipids" (fats) in your blood have been reduced to a normal concentration • many tobacco-related, white patches in your mouth have disappeared
Within 9 months *(for pregnant women)*	• your risk of experiencing pregnancy complications or fetal death has returned to the level of a nonsmoker
Within 1 year	• your chances of developing heart disease have been reduced by 50% • your lungs have increased their ability to fight off infections • your risk of developing a peptic ulcer has lowered to that of a nonsmoker • your health complaints, illnesses, and medical bills have decreased
Within 18 months	• your lung cilia have completed their task of cleaning out the residual tars and poisons in your lungs
Within 5 years	• your probability of contracting mouth, throat, and esophageal cancer has been reduced by one-half • your risk of developing lung cancer has decreased by 50 percent
Within 10 years	• your chances of becoming a victim of lung cancer have decreased by 30 to 50 percent, as compared to smokers
Within 15 years	• your likelihood of having a heart attack has become equal to that of a nonsmoker

Quitting is a process, not a single event. The 1988 Surgeon General's Report has shown that multiple attempts to quit actually increase the chances for long-term success.

Becoming an Ex-Tobacco User

There is no "best way" to quit using tobacco, and every known method can claim a certain degree of success. Many smokers want a short-cut to cessation, but it does not exist. The physiological, psychological, and social payoffs of smoking are not easily given up. However, when the desire is strong—a way will be found. Behavioral change is a crucial part of cessation. Take time to plan your coping strategies in advance.

Here are a few guidelines that may help.

- Set your quit date far enough in the future to allow for mental preparation, but not so distant that it will allow you to procrastinate. A good time is right after you have had your teeth professionally cleaned.

- Taper off from tobacco use, and your nicotine levels will drop gradually, lessening the severity of your withdrawal symptoms.

- The cold turkey method—stopping completely—all at once is the method most smokers (about 80%) use to quit. Nicotine levels drop quickly after quitting, and withdrawal symptoms can be intense—especially for the first 3-4 days. However, many individuals get over the discomfort of physical withdrawal within a week.

- Make two lists: the risks of continuing your tobacco use, and the benefits of quitting. Review them from time to time.

Choosing a Cessation Program

While many individuals are able to succeed alone via "cold turkey" quitting, you may need the support and encouragement provided by individualized or group cessation programs. These are offered by the American Cancer Society, American Lung Association, Seventh Day Adventists, and many local hospitals or wellness programs.

- Health care providers who have special training and experience in treating tobacco-related addictive and behavioral problems can also help if you are strongly addicted to tobacco. The more help you receive, the better your chances become of stopping for good.

- Nicotine-replacement therapy (the use of patches, gum, or nasal medications to ease the quitting process) can help you deal with the physical urges and cravings for nicotine. They are therapeutically designed to control nicotine dosages, and thus, to manage your cravings and withdrawal symptoms. Your resulting sense of calm and well-being will enable you to more successfully address the psychological and social aspects of your nicotine addiction. Less medication is needed as you progress through the stages of quitting. By continuing with your program, you can reach your tobacco-free goal in an additional 4–12 weeks.

- Ask your physician, dentist, or hygienist about using any of these aids. These agents have been thoroughly tested and approved by the Food and Drug Administration (FDA). The FDA continues to test new products as well.

- After determining; your own possible level of addiction to tobacco and readiness to quit, make improved oral health part of your cessation program.

Determine Your Degree of Addiction

By completing the following two tests, you can determine your degree of addiction to cigarette smoking.

The Fagerström Test for Nicotine Addiction

Questions	Answers (Points)
1. How soon after you wake do you smoke your first cigarette?	Within 5 minutes (3) 6-30 minutes (2)
2. Do you find it difficult to refrain from smoking in places where it is forbidden, eg, at the library, in church, at the theater?	Yes (1) No (0)
3. Which cigarette would you hate most to give up?	First one in the morning (1) All others (0)
4. How many cigarettes a day do you smoke?	10 or less (0) 11-20 (1) 21-30 (2) 31 or more (3)
5. Do you smoke more frequently during the first hours after waking than during the rest of the day?	Yes (1) No (0)
6. Do you smoke when you are so ill that you are in bed most of the day?	Yes (1) No (0)

If you score 6 points or more on this test, you may very well be addicted to nicotine. For assistance in quitting smoking, consult an oral health professional or physician.

The Smoker's (Horn) Self-Test

This test lists six psychological factors that contribute to ongoing cigarette use. Those who score 10 or above (out of a possible 15) on two or more of these factors are considered to be psychologically addicted to cigarettes.

	Always	Frequently	Occasionally	Seldom	Never
A. I smoke cigarettes to keep from slowing down	5	4	3	2	1
B. Handling a cigarette is part of the enjoyment of smoking	5	4	3	2	1
C. Smoking cigarettes is pleasant and relaxing	5	4	3	2	1
D. I light up a cigarette when I'm upset about something	5	4	3	2	1
E. When I run out of cigarettes, I find it almost unbearable	5	4	3	2	1
F. I smoke automatically without even being aware of it	5	4	3	2	1
G. I smoke to perk myself up	5	4	3	2	1
H. Part of the enjoyment of smoking comes from the steps I take to light up	5	4	3	2	1
I. I find cigarettes pleasurable	5	4	3	2	1
J. When I feel uncomfortable about something, I light up a cigarette	5	4	3	2	1
K. I am very much aware of the fact when I am not smoking	5	4	3	2	1
L. I light up a cigarette without realizing I still have one burning in the ashtray	5	4	3	2	1
M. I smoke to give myself a "lift"	5	4	3	2	1
N. Part of the enjoyment of smoking is in watching the smoke I exhale	5	4	3	2	1
O. I want a cigarette most when I am comfortable and relaxed	5	4	3	2	1
P. When I feel "blue" or want to take my mind off my cares, I smoke a cigarette	5	4	3	2	1
Q. I get a real craving for a cigarette when I haven't smoked for a while	5	4	3	2	1
R. I've found a cigarette in my mouth and didn't remember having put it there	5	4	3	2	1

Adding up your score

Use the following table to score yourself:

1. Enter your circled number for each statement in the space provided, putting the number for statement A on line A, for statement B on line B, and so on.

2. Add the three scores on each line (eg. the sum of your scores on lines A, G, and M gives yhou a total score for the "Stimulation" category).

A	+	G	+	M	=	Stimulation
B	+	H	+	N	=	Handling
C	+	I	+	O	=	Pleasure
D	+	J	+	P	=	Relaxation/Tension reduction
E	+	K	+	Q	=	Craving
F	+	L	+	R	=	Habit

A score of 10 more indicates an important reason. The higher your score (15 is the highest), the more important the reason. If you have a high score in more than one area, it may make quitting more difficult for you. When you know what you derive from smoking, you can look for satisfying substitutes.

Tips for Staying Tobacco Free

- Admit to yourself that you are addicted to tobacco. Don't tell yourself that one smoke, or chew, won't matter—it will.

- Take one day at a time. Don't decide to quit forever, just for today.

- Avoid tension-building situations. This is not the time to go on a crash diet or tackle a difficult problem.

- Stay well rested. Go to bed early every night during your withdrawal period.

- Brush or floss your teeth or use a mouthwash when you have the urge to use tobacco.

- Stay away from strong temptation, especially in the early stages of your recovery. Alcohol can weaken your resolve, so avoid drinking. Limit your contact with tobacco-using friends or relatives.

- Take six slow, deep breaths when you have the urge to smoke or use smokeless tobacco. Inhale strength and calmness, and exhale toxic poisons and feelings.

- Get adequate exercise. Stretch often, take a short walk, climb a flight of stairs.

- Remove all evidence of your addiction from your home, car, and workplace. Don't carry matches or a cigarette lighter.

- Drink water or fruit juice—fluid intake lessens cravings. However, avoid coffee or other beverages you associate with smoking or using smokeless tobacco.

- Reward yourself regularly for quitting. Save the money that you are not spending on tobacco and buy yourself a meaningful gift.

- Ask your dentist, physician, or pharmacist about using nicotine-replacement therapy products, and follow his or her professional advice.

- Increase your support system. Enlist your family, friends, coworkers, and/or health care providers to give you ongoing support.

- You don't fail if you have a slip or a relapse, but only if you don't keep trying to quit.

- Call a supportive friend when you feel the need to use tobacco. Share your feelings with this person.

- Tell others that you are quitting and encourage someone else to quit. This will make you more accountable.

- Find ways to handle stressful situations without a "nicotine fix." Never get too hungry, angry, lonely, or tired. These emotional states can lead you right back to tobacco use.

- If you relapse, immediately identify the cause of your slip, and plan to cope with this problem more effectively in the future.